10-Day Health Transformation

10-Day Health Transformation

Simple Steps to a Vibrant Life

Ava Michelle

COPYRIGHT PAGE

TABLE OF CONTENT

CHAPTER ONE
Setting the Stage for a Health Transformation Journey

1.1 Importance of Taking Charge of your Health

In today's fast-paced and demanding world, it is easy to overlook the most valuable asset we possess: our health. The hustle and bustle of daily life often leads us to neglect our well-being, as we prioritize work, responsibilities, and external obligations. However, it is crucial to recognize the profound importance of taking charge of our health. By assuming responsibility for our physical, mental, and emotional well-being, we embark on a transformative journey towards a better and more fulfilling life.

Taking charge of our health empowers us to become active participants in our own lives. It means accepting that our well-being is our responsibility and that our choices significantly impact our overall health. By acknowledging this fact, we reclaim control over our lives, making informed decisions that promote our physical fitness, mental clarity, and emotional resilience.

Proactively managing our health allows us to focus on prevention rather than reacting to health issues when they arise. By adopting healthy habits and lifestyle choices, we can minimize the risk of developing chronic diseases and promote longevity. Regular exercise, a balanced diet, adequate sleep, and stress management techniques are all essential components of preventive care. Additionally, by being proactive, we can detect early warning signs of potential health problems and seek medical intervention promptly, increasing the likelihood of successful treatment and recovery.

Optimal health directly impacts our quality of life. When we take charge of our health, we experience enhanced energy levels, increased vitality, and improved mental clarity. Physical fitness enables us to engage in activities we enjoy, fostering a sense of fulfillment and accomplishment. Moreover, good health positively influences our relationships, as we have the energy and emotional well-being to connect and engage with others on a deeper level.

Neglecting our health can have dire consequences not only for our well-being but also for our financial stability. By taking charge of our health, we reduce the likelihood of developing chronic conditions that require extensive medical intervention and long-term care. This proactive approach can lead to a significant reduction in healthcare costs, allowing us to allocate our resources towards other aspects of our lives, such as personal growth, education, or experiences.

When we prioritize our health, we become role models for those around us, especially family members and friends. By demonstrating a commitment to self-care, we inspire others to follow suit, creating a ripple effect of positive change. Taking charge of our health enables us to become agents of influence, encouraging loved ones to adopt healthy habits and embark on their own transformative journeys.

Taking charge of our health is not a luxury but a fundamental necessity. It empowers us to reclaim control over our lives, prioritize prevention, and enhance our overall well-being. By assuming responsibility for our health, we embark on a journey that leads to a better quality of life, reduced healthcare costs, and the ability to positively influence those around us. Let us recognize the importance of our health and commit to the self-care practices that will propel us towards a more vibrant and fulfilling existence.

1.2 Overview of the 10-day Transformation Program

In the pursuit of a healthier and more vibrant life, many individuals seek transformative programs that provide a structured and focused approach to well-being. The 10-Day Transformation Program is designed to offer individuals a comprehensive and actionable plan to kick start their journey towards improved health. By incorporating key principles such as nutrition, exercise, mindfulness, and self-care, this program aims to provide a holistic approach to wellness within a condensed timeframe.

1. Setting Clear Goals: The first step of the 10-Day Transformation Program is to set clear and realistic goals. Participants are encouraged to define their desired outcomes, whether it be weight loss, increased energy, improved mental clarity, or overall well-being. These goals serve as a compass throughout the program, providing focus and motivation.

2. Nutrition for Optimal Health: A significant aspect of the program revolves around nutrition. Participants are guided to adopt a healthy eating plan that emphasizes whole, unprocessed foods while minimizing or eliminating processed foods, refined sugars, and artificial additives. The program may include a specific meal plan or guidelines to follow, ensuring participants receive adequate nutrients while supporting their health goals.

3. Exercise and Movement: Physical activity is another crucial element of the 10-Day Transformation Program. Participants are encouraged to engage in regular exercise that suits their fitness level and preferences. This may include a combination of cardiovascular exercises, strength training, flexibility exercises, or activities like yoga or Pilates. The program emphasizes the importance of incorporating movement into daily routines to promote overall fitness and vitality.

4. Mindfulness and Self-Care: The program recognizes the essential role of mental and emotional well-being in overall health. Participants are introduced to mindfulness practices, stress management techniques, and self-care rituals. This may involve meditation, deep breathing exercises, journaling, or engaging in activities that promote relaxation and self-reflection. By nurturing the mind and emotions, individuals can enhance their overall well-being and resilience.

5. Detoxification and Cleansing: The 10-Day Transformation Program often incorporates a detoxification phase. This may involve specific dietary protocols or the inclusion of natural detoxifying agents. Detoxification aims to support the body's natural detox pathways and eliminate toxins that may hinder optimal health. This phase is typically followed by a transition to a sustainable and balanced diet.

6. Support and Accountability: A key feature of the program is the provision of support and accountability mechanisms. Participants may have access to a supportive community, online forums, or a designated coach who can guide and motivate them throughout the journey. This support system fosters a sense of camaraderie, enabling participants to share experiences, seek guidance, and celebrate milestones together.

Benefits of the 10-Day Transformation Program

The 10-Day Transformation Program offers several benefits to participants:

1. Kick-start to a Healthier Lifestyle: The program provides a structured and time-bound approach that jumpstarts individuals towards adopting healthier habits.

2. Increased Awareness: Participants gain a deeper understanding of the impact of nutrition, exercise, mindfulness, and self-care on their overall well-being.

3. Tangible Results: The condensed timeframe of the program allows individuals to witness tangible improvements in their energy levels, weight, mental clarity, and overall vitality.

4. Motivation and Momentum: The program creates a positive momentum and motivation for individuals to continue their wellness journey beyond the initial 10 days.

5. Education and Empowerment: Participants acquire knowledge, tools, and strategies that empower them to make informed decisions about their health long after the program concludes.

The 10-Day Transformation Program offers individuals a comprehensive and actionable plan to improve their health and well-being. By focusing on nutrition, exercise, mindfulness, and self-care, this program empowers participants to make positive changes within a condensed timeframe. Through goal setting, support systems, and a holistic approach, individuals can experience tangible improvements, increased awareness, and the motivation to continue their wellness journey beyond the 10 days. The program serves as a catalyst for transformative change, providing participants with the tools and knowledge necessary to embrace a healthier and more vibrant life.

1.3 Exploring the mind-body connection

The mind and body have long been viewed as separate entities, with distinct functions and influences. However, a growing body of research and ancient wisdom suggests a profound interconnection between the two. The mind-body connection refers to the intricate relationship between our thoughts, emotions, beliefs, and physical well-being.

The mind and body are not isolated entities but intricately intertwined aspects of human existence. The mind encompasses our thoughts, beliefs, emotions, and consciousness, while the body encompasses our physical structure, physiological processes, and sensations. The mind and body constantly interact and influence each other, forming a dynamic and complex relationship.

Our thoughts and beliefs have a profound impact on our physical well-being. Positive thoughts and optimistic beliefs can promote healing, enhance resilience, and boost overall health. Conversely, negative thoughts, stress, and limiting beliefs can contribute to the development of physical ailments, weaken the immune system, and hinder the body's natural healing processes.

Emotions play a crucial role in the mind-body connection. Unresolved emotional issues, such as chronic stress, anxiety, or unresolved trauma, can manifest as physical symptoms and illnesses. Emotional well-being and self-awareness are vital for maintaining a healthy mind-body balance. Practices such as mindfulness, meditation, and therapy can help individuals develop emotional resilience and foster a harmonious connection between the mind and body.

The stress response is a prime example of the mind-body connection in action. When we experience stress, whether physical or psychological, our body releases stress hormones such as cortisol and adrenaline. Prolonged or chronic stress can lead to adverse health effects, including cardiovascular problems, compromised immune function, digestive issues, and mental health disorders. Managing stress through relaxation techniques, exercise, and self-care is crucial for maintaining a healthy mind-body balance.

The mind's influence on the body is exemplified by the placebo and nocebo effects. Placebos, inert substances or treatments, can elicit positive health outcomes simply because the individual believes they are receiving a beneficial intervention. Conversely, the nocebo effect occurs when negative beliefs or expectations result in adverse effects, even with inert substances. These phenomena demonstrate the mind's remarkable ability to influence physical responses.

Mind-body practices provide practical avenues to nurture the mind-body connection. Techniques such as yoga, Tai Chi, Qigong, and meditation integrate physical movement, breath-work, and mental focus to promote overall well-being. These practices facilitate relaxation, reduce stress, enhance self-awareness, and cultivate a harmonious connection between the mind and body.

Implications for Health and Well-being

1. Holistic Approach to Healing: Recognizing the mind-body connection encourages a holistic approach to health and healing. Addressing physical symptoms alone may provide temporary relief, but a comprehensive approach that considers emotional, mental, and spiritual aspects promotes long-lasting well-being.

2. Self-Care and Stress Management: Nurturing the mind-body connection underscores the importance of self-care and stress management practices. Engaging in activities that promote relaxation, mindfulness, and emotional well-being supports a healthy mind-body balance and enhances overall health.

3. Integrative Medicine: The mind-body connection has led to the emergence of integrative medicine, which combines conventional medical treatments with complementary and alternative approaches that support the mind-body connection. This holistic approach recognizes the interconnectedness of all aspects of health.

Exploring the mind-body connection reveals a profound relationship between our thoughts, emotions, beliefs, and physical well-being.

Understanding and nurturing this connection can have far-reaching implications for our health and well-being. By recognizing the power of our thoughts, managing stress, and embracing mind-body practices, we can cultivate a harmonious and balanced relationship between our minds and bodies. The mind-body connection invites us to embark on a journey of self-discovery, self-care, and holistic healing, ultimately leading to a more vibrant and fulfilling life.

CHAPTER TWO
Assessing Your Current Health Status

2.1 Evaluating your lifestyle and habits

Our lifestyle and habits play a significant role in shaping our overall well-being and quality of life. They influence our physical health, mental and emotional state, relationships, productivity, and fulfillment. It is essential to regularly evaluate our lifestyle and habits to identify areas that may require improvement and make informed choices that align with our values and goals.

Evaluating our lifestyle and habits fosters self-awareness, enabling us to understand how our choices and behaviors impact our lives. This process allows us to reflect on our values, aspirations, and priorities, encouraging personal growth and self-improvement. By gaining a deeper understanding of ourselves, we can make intentional choices that support our well-being and align with our long-term goals.

Our lifestyle and habits directly influence our physical health. Evaluating our eating patterns, exercise routines, sleep habits, and self-care practices helps us identify areas for improvement. It enables us to make healthier choices, such as adopting a balanced diet, engaging in regular physical activity, getting sufficient sleep, and managing stress effectively. These changes can lead to increased energy levels, improved immune function, enhanced vitality, and reduced risk of chronic diseases.

Lifestyle and habits significantly impact our mental and emotional well-being. Evaluating factors such as stress levels, time management, social connections, and leisure activities can help us identify sources of stress or imbalance. It allows us to make adjustments that promote mental clarity, emotional resilience, and a sense of fulfillment. This may involve practicing mindfulness, engaging in activities that bring joy and relaxation, seeking support when needed, and cultivating healthy relationships.

Our habits and lifestyle choices also influence our productivity and time management skills. Assessing how we allocate our time, prioritize tasks, and manage distractions can reveal areas for improvement. By optimizing our routines, setting clear goals, and implementing effective time management strategies, we can enhance our productivity, accomplish more meaningful tasks, and create a sense of balance in our lives.

Our lifestyle and habits impact our relationships and social connections. Evaluating how we communicate, spend time with loved ones, and nurture connections can help us identify areas where we can enhance our relationships. This may involve active listening, effective communication skills, quality time spent with loved ones, and fostering a supportive network of friends and family.

Practical Strategies for Evaluating and Implementing Positive Change

1. Self-Reflection and Assessment: Take time for self-reflection and introspection. Assess different areas of your life, such as health, relationships, career, and personal growth. Identify strengths and areas that require improvement.

2. Goal Setting: Set specific, measurable, achievable, relevant, and time-bound (SMART) goals based on your assessment. Break down larger goals into smaller, actionable steps that can be implemented gradually.

3. Keep a Journal: Maintain a journal to track your daily habits and routines. Note your thoughts, emotions, activities, and behaviors. This practice can help you identify patterns, triggers, and areas for improvement.

4. Seek Feedback and Support: Reach out to trusted friends, family members, or mentors for feedback and support. They can provide valuable insights, accountability, and encouragement throughout your journey of change.

5. Implement Incremental Changes: Start by making small, manageable changes to your lifestyle and habits. Focus on one or two areas at a time to avoid feeling overwhelmed. Celebrate even the smallest successes to stay motivated.

6. Practice Mindfulness and Reflection: Cultivate mindfulness and engage in regular reflection. This can help you stay attuned to your thoughts, emotions, and behaviors, facilitating conscious decision-making and positive habit formation.

Regularly evaluating our lifestyle and habits is a powerful tool for personal growth, well-being, and self-improvement. By becoming aware of our choices, we can align our lifestyles with our values, goals, and aspirations. Evaluating our physical health, mental and emotional well-being, productivity, and relationships empowers us to make intentional changes that enhance our overall quality of life. Through self-reflection, goal setting, and incremental changes, we can embark on a transformative journey towards a more fulfilling and balanced existence.

2.2 Identifying areas of improvement

Continuous personal growth and development are essential aspects of a fulfilling and successful life. To embark on this journey, it is crucial to identify areas of improvement in our lives. Recognizing areas that require attention and growth enables us to make intentional changes, overcome obstacles, and unlock our true potential.

Self-reflection is a powerful tool for identifying areas of improvement. By taking the time to introspect and evaluate ourselves, we gain a deeper understanding of our strengths, weaknesses, values, and aspirations. This self-awareness allows us to recognize patterns, habits, and behaviors that may hinder our personal growth. Through introspection, we can pinpoint areas in which we can grow and develop.

Identifying areas of improvement involves aligning our goals and actions with our personal values. By clarifying our values, we can assess whether our current lifestyle, behaviors, and choices align with what truly matters to us. This process helps us identify any discrepancies and recognize areas where we can make changes that align more closely with our values and aspirations.

Seeking feedback from trusted individuals, such as mentors, friends, or colleagues, can provide valuable insights and perspectives on areas of improvement. External viewpoints can shed light on blind spots, highlight areas where we can enhance our skills or attitudes, and offer suggestions for growth. Welcoming constructive criticism and feedback opens doors to personal and professional development.

Regularly assessing our personal and professional growth is essential to identify areas of improvement. This may involve evaluating our skills, knowledge, achievements, and challenges in various domains of life, such as career, relationships, health, and personal development. Reflecting on our progress helps us identify areas where we can enhance our abilities, broaden our knowledge, or address specific weaknesses.

Developing emotional intelligence is key to identifying areas of improvement. Emotional self-awareness allows us to recognize patterns of behavior, triggers, and emotional responses that may hinder our personal growth. By cultivating emotional intelligence and self-management skills, we can identify areas where we can improve our communication, relationships, self-regulation, and decision-making abilities.

Practical Strategies for Identifying Areas of Improvement

1. Self-Assessment and Goal Setting: Engage in self-assessment exercises to evaluate different areas of your life. Consider your goals, values, and aspirations. Set specific and measurable goals for improvement in these areas, focusing on one or two at a time.

2. Seek Diverse Perspectives: Surround yourself with diverse individuals and seek their perspectives on areas of improvement. Engage in open and honest conversations, seek feedback, and be receptive to different viewpoints. This can provide valuable insights and help you gain new perspectives.

3. Embrace Continuous Learning: Commit to a mindset of continuous learning and growth. Seek opportunities for personal and professional development, such as attending workshops, courses, or seminars. Expand your knowledge, acquire new skills, and stay updated in your field of interest.

4. Embrace Challenges and Take Risks: Stepping out of your comfort zone and embracing challenges is crucial for personal growth. Take calculated risks and seize opportunities that stretch your abilities. Embracing challenges allows you to learn from failures, overcome obstacles, and discover new strengths and abilities.

5. Regular Reflection and Adjustment: Set aside time for regular reflection and evaluation of your progress. Assess whether you are moving closer to your goals and identify areas where adjustments are needed. Celebrate successes, acknowledge setbacks, and adjust your strategies accordingly.

Identifying areas of improvement is a vital step towards personal growth, self-actualization, and success. Through self-reflection, goal alignment, feedback, and continuous learning, we can identify areas where we can enhance our skills, attitudes, and behaviors. Embracing challenges, seeking diverse perspectives, and engaging in regular reflection empower us to make positive changes and reach our full potential. By identifying areas of improvement and taking proactive steps towards growth, we embark on a journey of self-discovery and transformation that leads to a more fulfilling and successful life.

2.3 Conducting health assessments and measurements

Health assessments and measurements serve as valuable tools in evaluating and monitoring our overall well-being. They provide objective insights into our physical, mental, and emotional health, allowing us to identify potential areas of concern, track progress, and make informed decisions about our lifestyle and healthcare choices.

Health assessments encompass a holistic evaluation of various aspects of our well-being. They involve gathering data and information related to physical health, mental and emotional state, lifestyle habits, medical history, and family background. By conducting a comprehensive health evaluation, we can obtain a comprehensive picture of our overall health and identify potential risk factors or areas that require attention.

Objective health measurements provide quantifiable data that help us assess and track our health status. These measurements can include body mass index (BMI), blood pressure, cholesterol levels, blood sugar levels, heart rate, and other relevant parameters. By obtaining these measurements, we can identify any deviations from healthy ranges, monitor progress, and make targeted interventions to improve our health.

Health assessments and measurements play a crucial role in early detection and prevention of diseases. Regular screenings, such as mammograms, Pap smears, prostate exams, and blood tests, can help identify potential health issues at an early stage when they are most treatable. Early detection allows for timely interventions, potentially preventing the progression of diseases and promoting better health outcomes.

Conducting health assessments and measurements enables us to track our progress and measure the effectiveness of interventions or lifestyle changes. By regularly evaluating our health markers, we can observe improvements, identify areas that still require attention, and stay motivated on our wellness journey. Seeing tangible results can boost our confidence, reinforce positive behaviors, and inspire further positive changes.

Health assessments provide personalized insights into our unique health needs and risks. By understanding our individual health profile, we can tailor our approach to health management. This may involve modifying our diet, adopting appropriate exercise regimens, managing stress levels, and seeking targeted medical interventions or therapies. Personalized health management improves the effectiveness of our efforts and enhances overall well-being.

Practical Strategies for Conducting Health Assessments and Measurements

1. Establish Baseline Measurements: Start by establishing baseline measurements of key health markers. This may include obtaining baseline weight, body measurements, blood pressure, cholesterol levels, and other relevant parameters. These baseline measurements serve as reference points for future assessments and comparisons.

2. Regular Health Screenings: Schedule regular health screenings based on age, gender, and individual risk factors. Consult with healthcare professionals to determine the appropriate screenings for your specific needs. Regular screenings help identify potential issues early on and enable timely interventions.

3. Utilize Technology and Apps: Take advantage of technology and health-tracking apps to assist in conducting and monitoring health assessments and measurements. These tools can help you record and track data such as physical activity, sleep patterns, heart rate, calorie intake, and other relevant health metrics.

4. Consult Healthcare Professionals: Seek guidance from healthcare professionals, such as physicians, nutritionists, or fitness trainers, who can provide expert advice on conducting health assessments and measurements. They can assist in interpreting results, offering personalized recommendations, and monitoring progress.

5. Maintain Health Records: Keep a record of your health assessments and measurements over time. This allows for easy comparison, tracking progress, and identifying trends or patterns. Maintain a dedicated health journal or utilize electronic health record systems for organized documentation.

Conducting health assessments and measurements is a vital step in understanding and improving our overall well-being. By gathering objective data, identifying potential health risks, and tracking progress, we can make informed decisions and take proactive steps towards better health. Regular assessments enable early detection, prevention, and personalized health management, contributing to long-term well-being and quality of life. By embracing health assessments and measurements as a regular practice, we empower ourselves to prioritize our health, make targeted interventions, and lead healthier, happier lives.

CHAPTER THREE
Setting Goals for Your Transformation

3.1 Establishing realistic and achievable health goals

Setting health goals is a powerful strategy for improving our well-being and leading a fulfilling life. However, it is crucial to establish goals that are realistic and achievable to maintain motivation and sustain long-term progress. By setting attainable health goals, we can create a roadmap for success, develop healthy habits, and experience positive transformations.

Establishing realistic and achievable health goals provides a solid foundation for sustainable well-being. It allows us to set clear intentions and define the path we wish to embark on. By outlining achievable goals, we lay the groundwork for gradual, consistent progress, avoiding the pitfalls of unrealistic expectations that can lead to frustration or burnout.

Realistic and achievable health goals help to maintain motivation and commitment over time. When goals are within our reach, we experience a sense of accomplishment and satisfaction as we make progress. This positive reinforcement fuels our motivation, empowering us to continue striving towards our objectives and sustaining long-term behavior change.

Establishing realistic health goals enables us to build sustainable and healthy habits. By breaking down larger goals into smaller, manageable steps, we create a roadmap for developing consistent behaviors. Over time, these behaviors become ingrained as habits, contributing to lasting lifestyle changes that support our well-being.

Realistic and achievable health goals provide opportunities for tracking and celebrating progress. By setting measurable objectives, we can monitor our advancements and adjust our strategies accordingly. Regularly assessing and acknowledging our progress serves as a source of motivation, reinforcing positive habits and inspiring continued effort.

Realistic health goals promote a balanced approach to well-being. They take into account various aspects of our lives, such as physical fitness, nutrition, sleep, stress management, and mental health. By setting goals that consider these different dimensions, we ensure a comprehensive approach to our health and well-being.

Practical Strategies for Establishing Realistic and Achievable Health Goals

1. Assess Your Current Health Status: Begin by assessing your current health status across different areas, such as physical fitness, nutrition, and mental well-being. Reflect on areas that require improvement and identify specific objectives within each domain.

2. Break-Down Goals into Manageable Steps: Divide larger goals into smaller, actionable steps. This approach helps to prevent overwhelm and allows for incremental progress. Focus on one step at a time, celebrating achievements along the way.

3. Prioritize and Focus: Prioritize your health goals and focus on a few key objectives at a time. Trying to accomplish too much at once can lead to frustration and decreased motivation. Concentrate your efforts on the most critical areas and gradually expand from there.

4. Seek Professional Guidance: Consult with healthcare professionals, such as physicians, dietitians, or personal trainers, for expert guidance and support. They can assist in setting realistic goals, providing personalized recommendations, and offering accountability throughout your journey.

5. Develop Action Plans: Create detailed action plans for each goal, outlining specific steps, resources, and timelines. Break down the tasks needed to achieve your objectives, making them more manageable and actionable.

6. Regularly Assess and Adjust: Regularly assess your progress towards your health goals. Reflect on what is working well and what may need adjustment. Be flexible and adaptable, making modifications to your plans as necessary to ensure continued progress.

Establishing realistic and achievable health goals is vital for sustainable well-being. By setting goals that are within our reach, we build a solid foundation for progress, maintain motivation, and develop healthy habits.

With a balanced approach, measurable objectives, and a focus on continuous improvement, we pave the way for positive transformations and long-term success. By embracing these strategies and committing to realistic health goals, we empower ourselves to lead healthier, happier lives.

3.2 Defining success criteria for the 10-day transformation

The 10-Day Transformation program offers a unique opportunity for individuals to embark on a journey of personal growth, wellness, and transformation. To make the most of this program, it is crucial to define clear success criteria that align with our goals and aspirations. By establishing measurable benchmarks and criteria for success, we can track progress, stay motivated, and experience the full benefits of the transformation process.

Defining success criteria for the 10-Day Transformation provides clarity and focus on what we hope to achieve. It allows us to set specific, measurable goals that guide our actions and keep us on track throughout the program. By clearly defining our desired outcomes, we establish a clear vision of success.

Success is subjective and unique to each individual. Defining success criteria allows us to personalize our goals and outcomes based on our individual needs, desires, and aspirations. It enables us to align the transformation process with our specific definition of success, enhancing our motivation and sense of fulfillment.

Setting success criteria creates a sense of motivation and accountability. By establishing specific milestones and benchmarks, we hold ourselves accountable to our goals and commitments. This accountability serves as a driving force to stay committed to the program and make consistent progress.

Defining success criteria provides a means to track our progress and evaluate the effectiveness of the 10-Day Transformation. By establishing measurable benchmarks, we can assess our achievements, identify areas of improvement, and make necessary adjustments to our approach. Regular evaluation allows us to fine-tune our strategies and optimize our results.

Clearly defined success criteria allow us to celebrate milestones and achievements along the way. By breaking down the transformation process into smaller, achievable goals, we create opportunities for celebration and reinforcement. Celebrating these milestones fuels our motivation, boosts our confidence, and encourages continued progress.

Practical Strategies for Defining Success Criteria

1. Align Success Criteria with Personal Values: Consider your personal values and priorities when defining success criteria. Reflect on how the transformation program aligns with your core values and aspirations. This alignment ensures that your success criteria resonate deeply with your sense of purpose and fulfillment.

2. Establish Short-Term and Long-Term Milestones: Break down the transformation process into short-term and long-term milestones. This allows you to track progress and experience a sense of accomplishment along the way. Short-term milestones can act as stepping stones towards achieving your long-term goals.

3. Consider Multiple Dimensions of Wellness: Define success criteria that encompass multiple dimensions of wellness, including physical, mental, emotional, and social aspects. This holistic approach ensures a well-rounded transformation experience and promotes overall well-being.

4. Regularly Evaluate and Adjust: Regularly evaluate your progress against the defined success criteria. Assess your achievements, challenges, and areas of improvement. Make necessary adjustments to your strategies or goals to stay aligned with your desired outcomes.

Defining success criteria for the 10-Day Transformation program is a crucial step in maximizing its benefits and achieving personal growth and wellness. By establishing clear and measurable benchmarks, we gain focus, motivation, and accountability. These success criteria allow us to track progress, celebrate achievements, and make necessary adjustments along the way. With a personalized and holistic approach to success, we set ourselves up for a transformative experience that aligns with our individual goals and aspirations. Embrace the power of defining success criteria, and unlock the full potential of the 10-Day Transformation journey.

3.3 Creating a vision for a vibrant life

Creating a vision for a vibrant life is an empowering and transformative process that allows individuals to define their dreams, aspirations, and desired outcomes. It involves envisioning a future that is filled with joy, purpose, and fulfillment. By crafting a clear and compelling vision, individuals can set the course for their lives, make intentional choices, and pursue a path that leads to a vibrant and meaningful existence.

Creating a vision for a vibrant life provides clarity and direction. It helps us define what we truly want in life, identify our passions and values, and articulate our deepest desires. With a clear vision, we gain a sense of purpose and a roadmap to guide our decisions, actions, and priorities.

A vibrant life vision serves as a constant source of motivation and inspiration. It ignites our inner drive, propelling us forward even in the face of challenges and setbacks. When we have a compelling vision that excites and resonates with us, we become more resilient, determined, and focused on pursuing our dreams.

Creating a vision for a vibrant life allows us to align our aspirations with our core values. It enables us to live authentically and in accordance with what truly matters to us. When our vision reflects our values, we experience a deep sense of fulfillment and harmony, knowing that our actions and choices are in alignment with our true selves.

By crafting a vision for a vibrant life, we bring our dreams and goals into focus. It serves as a catalyst for manifestation, encouraging us to set specific goals, take intentional action, and overcome obstacles along the way. When we have a clear vision, we are more likely to make progress towards our aspirations and turn them into reality.

Creating a vision for a vibrant life empowers us to take ownership of our lives and embrace personal growth. It encourages us to step out of our comfort zones, expand our horizons, and continuously evolve as individuals. Pursuing our vision requires us to develop new skills, cultivate resilience, and embrace opportunities for self-improvement.

Practical Strategies for Creating a Vision for a Vibrant Life

1. Reflect on Your Passions and Values: Take time to reflect on your passions, interests, and values. Identify what brings you joy, fulfillment, and a sense of purpose. These insights will form the foundation of your vision for a vibrant life.

2. Visualize Your Ideal Life: Use visualization techniques to imagine and visualize your ideal life. Envision the different aspects of your life, such as relationships, career, health, personal growth, and lifestyle. Paint a vivid picture of what a vibrant life looks and feels like to you.

3. Create a Vision Board: Compile images, quotes, and symbols that represent your vision for a vibrant life. Create a vision board that visually depicts your aspirations. Place it somewhere visible as a daily reminder of your dreams and goals.

4. Develop an Action Plan: Develop a comprehensive action plan that outlines the steps you need to take to manifest your vision. Break down your goals into smaller milestones and create a timeline for achieving them. Regularly review and update your action plan to stay on track.

5. Seek Support and Accountability: Share your vision with trusted friends, family, or mentors who can provide support, guidance, and accountability. Surround yourself with individuals who uplift and encourage you to pursue your dreams.

Creating a vision for a vibrant life is a powerful process that sets the stage for a fulfilling and purpose-driven existence. By defining your dreams, aligning with your values, and taking intentional action, you can manifest a life that is vibrant, joyful, and deeply meaningful. Embrace the journey of crafting your vision, and let it guide you towards a life that is in harmony with your truest self.

CHAPTER FOUR
Nutrition for Optimal Health

4.1 Understanding the basics of a healthy diet

A healthy diet forms the cornerstone of overall well-being and vitality. It provides essential nutrients, supports optimal physical and mental function, and reduces the risk of chronic diseases. Understanding the basics of a healthy diet empowers individuals to make informed choices, develop sustainable eating habits, and enjoy the benefits of a nourishing lifestyle.

A healthy diet revolves around consuming nutrient-rich foods. These include fruits, vegetables, whole grains, lean proteins, healthy fats, and low-fat dairy products. Nutrient-dense foods provide essential vitamins, minerals, antioxidants, and dietary fiber necessary for optimal health and vitality.

Portion control and moderation are key elements of a healthy diet. It involves consuming appropriate portions of food to meet nutritional needs without overindulging. Balancing portion sizes ensures a healthy energy balance and prevents overeating, contributing to weight management and overall well-being.

Hydration is an essential component of a healthy diet. Drinking an adequate amount of water throughout the day supports various bodily functions, such as digestion, nutrient absorption, temperature regulation, and cognitive function. Aim for at least eight glasses of water per day, adjusting based on individual needs and activity levels.

A healthy diet emphasizes the importance of balanced macronutrients: carbohydrates, proteins, and fats. Carbohydrates provide energy, proteins support tissue repair and growth, and fats provide essential fatty acids. Opt for complex carbohydrates, lean proteins, and healthy fats to maintain a balanced diet.

Minimizing processed foods and added sugars is crucial for a healthy diet. Processed foods are often high in unhealthy fats, sodium, and added sugars, while providing limited nutritional value. Choose whole, unprocessed foods whenever possible and limit intake of sugary beverages, sweets, and processed snacks.

A healthy diet embraces variety and colorful food choices. Different fruits, vegetables, and whole grains provide a diverse range of nutrients, flavors, and textures. Aim to incorporate a rainbow of fruits and vegetables to ensure a wide spectrum of vitamins, minerals, and antioxidants.

Mindful eating is a fundamental aspect of a healthy diet. It involves paying attention to the sensory experience of eating, listening to internal hunger and satiety cues, and savoring each bite. By practicing mindful eating, individuals can foster a healthier relationship with food, promote better digestion, and prevent overeating.

Practical Strategies for a Healthy Diet

1. Meal Planning and Preparation: Plan and prepare meals in advance to ensure a balanced and nutritious diet. This allows for healthier food choices, portion control, and reduced reliance on convenience foods. Incorporate a variety of nutrient-rich ingredients and experiment with new recipes to keep meals exciting.

2. Read Food Labels: Develop the habit of reading food labels to understand the nutritional content of packaged foods. Pay attention to serving sizes, ingredients, and nutrient information, especially regarding added sugars, unhealthy fats, and sodium. Choose foods with minimal processing and fewer artificial additives.

3. Include Physical Activity: Complement a healthy diet with regular physical activity. Engage in activities you enjoy, such as walking, jogging, cycling, or participating in sports. Physical activity enhances overall health, supports weight management, and complements the benefits of a nutritious diet.

4. Seek Professional Guidance: Consult a registered dietitian or nutritionist for personalized guidance and support. They can provide tailored advice based on individual needs, preferences, and any specific dietary restrictions or health conditions.

Understanding the basics of a healthy diet is essential for nourishing the body and mind. By incorporating nutrient-rich foods, practicing portion control, staying hydrated, and minimizing processed foods and added sugars, we can cultivate a lifestyle that promotes optimal health and vitality. Embrace the principles of a healthy diet, make informed choices, and enjoy the journey of nourishing yourself through wholesome and balanced eating habits.

4.2 Exploring macronutrients and micronutrients

Macronutrients and micronutrients are essential components of our diet that play crucial roles in maintaining overall health and well-being. While macronutrients provide the body with energy, micronutrients are necessary for various physiological functions. Understanding the distinction between these two categories and their significance can empower individuals to make informed dietary choices and optimize their nutrition.

Macronutrients: Fueling the Body

Macronutrients are the nutrients required by the body in large quantities to provide energy and support various bodily functions. The three primary macronutrients are carbohydrates, proteins, and fats.

a. Carbohydrates: Carbohydrates are the body's main source of energy. They are found in foods such as grains, fruits, vegetables, and legumes. Carbohydrates can be classified as simple (found in sugary foods) or complex (found in whole grains and fiber-rich foods). They provide glucose, which fuels the brain, muscles, and other organs.

b. Proteins: Proteins are essential for growth, repair, and maintenance of body tissues, as well as the production of enzymes, hormones, and antibodies. Good sources of protein include lean meats, poultry, fish, eggs, dairy products, legumes, and plant-based sources like tofu and quinoa.

c. Fats: Fats are a concentrated source of energy and are involved in the absorption of fat-soluble vitamins. They also provide insulation and cushioning for organs. Healthy fat sources include nuts, seeds, avocados, olive oil, and fatty fish. It is important to choose unsaturated fats and limit saturated and trans-fats.

Micronutrients: Essential for Optimal Health

Micronutrients are nutrients required in smaller amounts but are equally important for the body's proper functioning. They include vitamins and minerals.

a. Vitamins: Vitamins are organic compounds that regulate various biochemical processes in the body. They play critical roles in metabolism, immune function, vision, bone health, and more. Vitamins are found in a variety of foods, such as fruits, vegetables, whole grains, dairy products, and lean proteins. Examples include vitamin C, vitamin D, vitamin B complex, and vitamin E.

b. Minerals: Minerals are inorganic substances necessary for various bodily functions, including bone health, nerve transmission, fluid balance, and enzyme activity. Examples of minerals include calcium, iron, potassium, magnesium, and zinc. Good sources of minerals include fruits, vegetables, whole grains, nuts, seeds, and dairy products.

Achieving a Balanced Diet

A balanced diet encompasses a proper combination of macronutrients and micronutrients to meet the body's nutritional needs. While macronutrients provide the energy required for daily activities, micronutrients support vital functions and help prevent nutrient deficiencies.

Achieving a balanced diet involves:

a. Varied Food Choices: Consume a variety of foods from different food groups to obtain a broad spectrum of nutrients.

b. Portion Control: Pay attention to portion sizes to maintain a healthy energy balance.

c. Whole, Unprocessed Foods: Focus on whole grains, lean proteins, healthy fats, fruits, and vegetables, which provide a wealth of macronutrients and micronutrients.

d. Nutrient Density: Choose nutrient-dense foods that provide a high amount of nutrients relative to their calorie content.

e. Adequate Hydration: Water is essential for overall health and aids in nutrient absorption and waste removal.

Macronutrients and micronutrients are vital components of a healthy and balanced diet. Understanding their roles, sources, and significance empowers individuals to make informed dietary choices and optimize their nutrition. By incorporating a variety of macronutrient-rich foods, along with a diverse range of micronutrient sources, we can nourish our bodies, support overall health, and enjoy the benefits of a well-rounded diet. Strive for a balanced and nutrient-dense approach to nutrition, and embrace the power of macronutrients and micronutrients for a healthier and more fulfilling life.

4.3 Designing a balanced meal plan for the 10-day transformation

Designing a balanced meal plan is a crucial aspect of the 10-Day Transformation program. A well-structured and nutrient-dense meal plan provides the foundation for achieving optimal health, supporting the body's needs, and promoting vibrant well-being. By carefully selecting and combining foods, individuals can create a meal plan that maximizes nutrient intake, supports energy levels, and facilitates the desired health transformation.

A balanced meal plan for the 10-Day Transformation should prioritize nutrient variety by incorporating a wide range of fruits, vegetables, whole grains, lean proteins, and healthy fats. Each meal should aim to include a variety of colors, textures, and flavors to ensure the intake of essential vitamins, minerals, antioxidants, and fiber. This variety supports overall health and helps meet the body's nutritional requirements.

Whole foods should form the basis of the meal plan, as they are minimally processed and retain their natural nutrients. Incorporate whole grains like quinoa, brown rice, and oats, along with fresh fruits, vegetables, legumes, and lean proteins such as poultry, fish, and plant-based sources like tofu and tempeh. Whole foods provide a rich array of macronutrients, micronutrients, and phytochemicals that support optimal health.

Portion control plays a vital role in maintaining energy balance and achieving desired health goals. Be mindful of portion sizes for each food group, ensuring that meals are balanced and appropriately sized. Include a mix of carbohydrates, proteins, and healthy fats in each meal, and use visual cues or measuring tools to gauge proper portion sizes. This approach helps prevent overeating and supports weight management.

A balanced meal plan should incorporate adequate amounts of carbohydrates, proteins, and fats. Carbohydrates provide energy, proteins support tissue repair and growth, and fats provide essential fatty acids. Include complex carbohydrates like whole grains, lean proteins, such as poultry, fish, beans, and lentils, and healthy fats from sources like avocados, nuts, and olive oil. This balanced macronutrient profile ensures sustained energy, satiety, and overall nutritional adequacy.

Incorporate mindful eating practices into the meal plan for the 10-Day Transformation. Slow down, savor each bite, and listen to your body's hunger and fullness cues. Avoid distractions during meals, such as screens or work, and focus on the sensory experience of eating. This mindful approach enhances digestion, improves nutrient absorption, and helps cultivate a healthier relationship with food.

Adequate hydration is essential for overall health and supports the body's detoxification processes. Include plenty of water throughout the day and consider incorporating hydrating foods such as cucumbers, watermelon, and citrus fruits. Avoid sugary beverages and prioritize water as the primary hydration source.

It is important to personalize the meal plan based on individual preferences, dietary restrictions, and specific health goals. Consider consulting a registered dietitian or nutritionist to tailor the meal plan to individual needs, ensuring nutritional adequacy and compatibility with the

10-Day Transformation program.

Designing a balanced meal plan for the 10-Day Transformation program is a key component of achieving optimal health and vitality. By prioritizing nutrient variety, practicing portion control, incorporating whole foods, and embracing mindful eating practices, individuals can create a meal plan that nourishes the body, supports energy levels, and promotes overall well-being. Personalize the plan based on individual needs and consult with professionals for guidance. Embrace the transformative power of a well-designed meal plan and experience the positive impact it can have on your health journey.

CHAPTER FIVE
Detoxifying Your Body

5.1 Importance of detoxification for overall health

Detoxification, often referred to as cleansing, is a process that supports the body's natural ability to eliminate toxins and waste products. In today's modern world, where we are exposed to various environmental pollutants, processed foods, and stressors, the importance of detoxification for overall health cannot be overstated. Detoxification helps optimize bodily functions, enhance well-being, and promote a balanced state of health.

Detoxification plays a vital role in eliminating harmful toxins and waste products that accumulate in the body. These toxins can come from external sources such as pollution, chemicals, pesticides, and heavy metals, as well as internal sources like metabolic byproducts and cellular waste. By supporting the body's detoxification pathways, we can reduce the burden of toxins and promote overall health.

Detoxification supports the optimal functioning of vital organs involved in the detoxification process, such as the liver, kidneys, lungs, skin, and digestive system. These organs work together to filter toxins, metabolize waste products, and eliminate them from the body. By supporting these organs' health and function, we ensure efficient detoxification and maintain overall well-being.

Detoxification can have a positive impact on digestive health. By eliminating toxins and supporting the digestive system, detoxification helps maintain a healthy gut environment, enhances nutrient absorption, and promotes regular bowel movements. This, in turn, reduces digestive discomfort, supports a balanced microbiome, and improves overall digestive function.

Detoxification can boost energy levels and enhance vitality. When the body is burdened with toxins, it can lead to fatigue, sluggishness, and reduced energy. By supporting the elimination of toxins and waste products, detoxification allows the body to operate more efficiently, leading to increased energy levels, improved mental clarity, and a greater sense of vitality.

A healthy and efficient detoxification process can strengthen the immune system. Toxins can impair immune function and make the body more susceptible to infections and diseases. By reducing the toxic load and supporting the elimination of waste products, detoxification helps bolster the immune system's ability to defend against pathogens and maintain overall health.

Detoxification not only benefits the physical body but also has a positive impact on mental and emotional well-being. Toxins can affect brain function, leading to brain fog, poor concentration, and mood imbalances. By supporting detoxification, we can experience improved mental clarity, enhanced cognitive function, and a greater sense of emotional balance.

Practical Ways to Support Detoxification

1. Hydration: Drink an adequate amount of water daily to support the elimination of toxins through the kidneys and promote overall hydration.

2. Nutrient-Dense Diet: Consume a diet rich in fruits, vegetables, whole grains, lean proteins, and healthy fats. These foods provide essential nutrients and antioxidants that support detoxification processes.

3. Avoid Toxins: Minimize exposure to environmental toxins by choosing organic foods, using natural cleaning and personal care products, and reducing exposure to pollutants.

4. Exercise: Engage in regular physical activity to stimulate circulation, promote lymphatic flow, and support the elimination of toxins through sweat.

5. Stress Management: Practice stress-reducing techniques such as meditation, deep breathing exercises, yoga, or mindfulness to support overall well-being and reduce the impact of stress on the body's detoxification processes.

Detoxification is a vital process for maintaining overall health and well-being in our modern world. By supporting the body's natural detoxification pathways, we can reduce the toxic burden, enhance organ function, improve digestive health, boost energy levels, strengthen the immune system, and promote mental and emotional well-being. Incorporating practical strategies to support detoxification, such as hydration, a nutrient-dense diet, toxin avoidance, regular exercise, and stress management, empowers individuals to take control of their health and enjoy the benefits of a cleansed body and revitalized mind. Embrace the importance of detoxification and embark on a journey toward a healthier and more vibrant life.

5.2 Detox methods and practices

Detoxification has become a popular topic in the realm of health and wellness, with numerous methods and practices aimed at supporting the body's natural cleansing process. Detox methods are designed to eliminate toxins, promote overall well-being, and restore balance to the body. It is important to note that individual experiences may vary, and it is advisable to consult with a healthcare professional before embarking on any detox program.

1. Dietary Approaches:

a. Whole Food Detox: This approach focuses on consuming whole, unprocessed foods and eliminating processed foods, added sugars, and artificial ingredients. It emphasizes fruits, vegetables, whole grains, lean proteins, healthy fats, and plenty of water.

b. Juice Cleanses: Juice cleanses involve consuming freshly pressed juices made from fruits and vegetables for a designated period. These cleanses provide a concentrated source of nutrients while allowing the digestive system to rest.

c. Elimination Diets: Elimination diets involve temporarily removing common allergens or inflammatory foods, such as gluten, dairy, or refined sugars, from the diet. This approach aims to identify and address potential food sensitivities or intolerances.

2. Hydration and Herbal Teas: Staying adequately hydrated is crucial for supporting the body's detoxification process. Drinking water helps flush out toxins and facilitates optimal organ function. Additionally, herbal teas, such as dandelion root, nettle, or ginger tea, may have detoxifying properties and support overall health.

3. Exercise and Sweat: Physical activity and sweating can aid in the detoxification process by promoting lymphatic flow and circulation. Engaging in regular exercise, such as cardiovascular activities, strength training, or yoga, can help eliminate toxins through sweat and support overall well-being.

4. Saunas and Steam Rooms: Saunas and steam rooms are often used as part of detoxification practices. These heated environments promote sweating and help eliminate toxins through the skin. They may also support relaxation and stress reduction.

5. Dry Brushing: Dry brushing involves using a natural bristle brush to gently massage the skin in circular motions. This practice helps exfoliate the skin, stimulate lymphatic drainage, and promote detoxification by removing dead skin cells and improving circulation.

6. Alternative Therapies:

a. Colon Hydrotherapy: Also known as colonic irrigation, this therapy involves gently flushing the colon with water to remove accumulated waste and toxins.

b. Liver Cleansing: Certain herbal supplements or dietary protocols are believed to support liver health and aid in detoxification processes. Milk thistle, dandelion root, and turmeric are commonly used herbs for liver support.

c. Ayurvedic Detoxification: Ayurveda, an ancient holistic healing system, includes practices such as oil pulling, herbal formulations, and specialized diets to support detoxification and restore balance.

7. Mindfulness Practices: Stress reduction and emotional well-being are essential aspects of detoxification. Mindfulness practices like meditation, deep breathing exercises, and yoga help reduce stress, promote relaxation, and support overall health.

Detox methods and practices aim to support the body's natural cleansing process and promote overall well-being. Dietary approaches, hydration, exercise, sweating, alternative therapies, and mindfulness practices are among the diverse range of methods individuals may consider. It is important to approach detoxification with caution, considering individual needs and consulting with healthcare professionals when necessary. By incorporating suitable detox methods and practices, individuals can support their bodies in eliminating toxins, restoring balance, and enjoying the benefits of enhanced well-being.

5.3 Implementing a detox plan during the transformation

During the transformation process, implementing a detox plan can be a valuable component of your journey towards improved health and well-being. A well-designed detox plan can help eliminate toxins, reset the body, and create a solid foundation for positive changes.

A detox plan allows you to clear toxins accumulated from environmental pollutants, processed foods, and lifestyle factors. By eliminating these toxins, you create a clean slate for your body to function optimally and absorb essential nutrients more efficiently.

Implementing a detox plan can help restore nutritional balance by emphasizing whole, nutrient-dense foods. By removing processed foods, artificial additives, and excessive sugars, you create space for nourishing your body with fresh fruits, vegetables, lean proteins, healthy fats, and whole grains. This supports cellular health, enhances energy levels, and promotes overall well-being.

A detox plan can revitalize your energy levels and promote a sense of vitality. By eliminating energy-draining processed foods and focusing on nutrient-dense options, you provide your body with the fuel it needs to thrive. Proper nutrition, along with the removal of toxins, can lead to increased energy, improved mental clarity, and a renewed sense of well-being.

Many detox plans emphasize foods that support digestive health, such as fiber-rich fruits and vegetables, fermented foods, and hydrating liquids. These dietary changes can promote regular bowel movements, support gut microbiome balance, and alleviate digestive discomfort. A healthy digestive system is essential for nutrient absorption and overall well-being.

Implementing a detox plan during the transformation can help strengthen the mind-body connection. By nourishing your body with wholesome foods and adopting healthy lifestyle practices, you create an environment conducive to mental clarity, emotional balance, and overall mindfulness. A clear and balanced body promotes a clear and balanced mind.

Practical Strategies for Successful Implementation

1. Set Clear Goals: Define your detox goals, whether it's reducing sugar intake, eliminating processed foods, or incorporating more plant-based meals. Having clear goals will guide your choices and help you stay focused during the transformation process.

2. Plan and Prepare: Take time to plan and prepare your detox plan. Create a meal plan that includes nutrient-rich foods, and stock your kitchen with wholesome ingredients. Preparing meals in advance can help you stay on track and avoid impulsive, unhealthy choices.

3. Hydration: Stay adequately hydrated during your detox plan. Drink plenty of water, herbal teas, and infused waters to support the elimination of toxins and maintain optimal hydration levels.

4. Mindful Eating: Practice mindful eating throughout your detox plan. Slow down, savor each bite, and pay attention to your body's hunger and fullness cues. This mindful approach promotes a deeper connection with your body's needs and enhances your overall dining experience.

5. Seek Support: Enlist the support of a friend, family member, or a health professional during your detox journey. Having someone to share your experiences, provide accountability, and offer guidance can make the process more enjoyable and sustainable.

Implementing a detox plan during the transformation is a powerful way to nurture your body and mind. By clearing toxins, restoring nutritional balance, boosting energy, supporting digestive health, and strengthening the mind-body connection, a well-designed detox plan can pave the way for long-lasting positive changes. Embrace the opportunity to reset your habits, prioritize wholesome foods, and adopt mindful practices. Remember that everyone's detox journey is unique, so listen to your body and make adjustments accordingly. Through the implementation of a thoughtfully designed detox plan, you can embark on a transformative path towards improved health and well-being.

CHAPTER SIX
Exercise and Movement

6.1 Benefits of regular physical activity

Regular physical activity is an essential component of a healthy lifestyle, offering a multitude of benefits for both the body and mind. Engaging in regular exercise and movement not only helps maintain physical fitness but also contributes to overall well-being.

Physical Health Benefits

a. Improved Cardiovascular Health: Regular exercise strengthens the heart and improves cardiovascular function, reducing the risk of heart disease, high blood pressure, and stroke. It helps lower bad cholesterol (LDL) levels and increases good cholesterol (HDL) levels.

b. Weight Management: Physical activity plays a crucial role in weight management and preventing obesity. Regular exercise helps burn calories, build muscle mass, and boost metabolism, promoting a healthy body composition.

c. Enhanced Bone and Joint Health: Weight-bearing exercises, such as walking, running, and strength training, contribute to stronger bones and reduce the risk of osteoporosis and fractures. Physical activity also helps maintain joint flexibility and reduces the likelihood of joint-related problems.

d. Increased Energy Levels: Engaging in regular physical activity improves stamina, increases oxygen and nutrient delivery to muscles, and enhances overall energy levels. Regular exercise has been shown to combat fatigue and promote a more active and energetic lifestyle.

Mental and Emotional Well-being Benefits

a. Stress Reduction: Physical activity is a natural stress reliever, triggering the release of endorphins, also known as "feel-good" hormones. Regular exercise helps reduce stress levels, alleviate anxiety and depression, and improve overall mood.

b. Improved Cognitive Function: Regular physical activity has been linked to improved cognitive function, including enhanced memory, concentration, and creativity. Exercise increases blood flow to the brain, promoting the growth of new neurons and improving cognitive performance.

c. Better Sleep Quality: Physical activity can positively impact sleep patterns and improve sleep quality. Regular exercise helps regulate the sleep-wake cycle, promotes relaxation, and reduces insomnia symptoms.

d. Boosted Self-esteem and Confidence: Engaging in regular physical activity fosters a sense of accomplishment, boosts self-esteem, and improves body image. Achieving fitness goals, experiencing progress, and feeling physically capable contribute to a positive self-perception.

e. Enhanced Mental Resilience: Regular exercise can improve mental resilience and coping skills, helping individuals better manage and navigate daily stressors. It promotes a sense of empowerment and fosters emotional well-being.

Longevity and Disease Prevention

a. Disease Prevention: Regular physical activity is associated with a reduced risk of chronic diseases such as cardiovascular disease, type 2 diabetes, certain cancers, and metabolic disorders. It supports a healthy immune system and reduces inflammation within the body.

b. Increased Longevity: Engaging in regular physical activity has been linked to increased life expectancy. Studies suggest that physically active individuals tend to have a lower risk of premature death compared to sedentary individuals.

c. Enhanced Quality of Life: Regular exercise improves overall quality of life by promoting physical independence, reducing the risk of functional limitations, and increasing overall vitality.

The benefits of regular physical activity extend beyond physical fitness, positively impacting mental, emotional, and overall well-being. By engaging in regular exercise, individuals can improve cardiovascular health, manage weight, strengthen bones and joints, boost energy levels, and promote longevity. Furthermore, physical activity supports mental and emotional well-being by reducing stress, enhancing cognitive function, improving sleep, and boosting self-esteem. Make regular physical activity a priority in your life, embracing the transformative power it has to nurture the body and mind, and experience the multitude of benefits it offers for a healthier and happier life.

6.2 Designing an exercise routine for the 10-day transformation

As part of the 10-day transformation, incorporating an exercise routine can significantly contribute to your overall well-being and maximize the benefits of the program. A well-designed exercise routine helps improve cardiovascular health, increase strength and endurance, enhance flexibility, and support mental and emotional well-being.

1. Assess Your Fitness Level and Goals:

Before designing an exercise routine, assess your current fitness level and determine your goals for the 10-day transformation. Are you looking to improve cardiovascular fitness, build strength, increase flexibility, or all of the above? Understanding your starting point and setting clear goals will help tailor the exercise routine to your specific needs.

2. Choose a Variety of Exercise Modalities:

Incorporate a variety of exercise modalities to engage different muscle groups, prevent boredom, and promote overall fitness. Include cardiovascular exercises (such as walking, jogging, cycling, or swimming) to improve heart health, strength training exercises (using bodyweight or resistance) to build lean muscle, and flexibility exercises (such as yoga or stretching) to enhance range of motion and promote relaxation.

3. Consider Time and Intensity:

Take into account the time available for exercise during the 10-day transformation and determine the intensity level that suits your fitness level and goals. Aim for at least 150 minutes of moderate-intensity aerobic activity or 75 minutes of vigorous-intensity aerobic activity per week, as recommended by health guidelines. Gradually increase the intensity of your workouts as your fitness level improves.

4. Warm-Up and Cool-Down:

Prioritize a proper warm-up and cool-down in your exercise routine. Begin each session with a few minutes of dynamic stretching or low-intensity movements to prepare your muscles for the upcoming workout. Afterward, cool down with static stretching and gentle movements to promote recovery and prevent muscle soreness.

5. Incorporate Strength Training:

Strength training exercises are crucial for building muscle, improving metabolism, and increasing overall strength and endurance. Include exercises that target major muscle groups, such as squats, lunges, push-ups, and planks. Start with lighter weights or bodyweight exercises and gradually progress to heavier weights or increased resistance as your fitness level allows.

6. Focus on Core Stability:

Core stability exercises, such as planks, bridges, and abdominal exercises, are essential for a strong and stable core. A strong core supports proper posture, reduces the risk of injury, and enhances overall functional fitness. Include core exercises in your routine to improve stability and balance.

7. Allow for Rest and Recovery:

While exercise is important, it is equally crucial to allow for proper rest and recovery. Schedule rest days throughout the 10-day transformation to give your body time to repair and rebuild. Listen to your body and adjust your exercise routine if you experience excessive fatigue or discomfort.

8. Stay Hydrated and Practice Proper Nutrition:

Hydration and proper nutrition are key components of any exercise routine. Drink water before, during, and after exercise to stay adequately hydrated. Additionally, support your workouts with a balanced diet that provides the necessary nutrients for energy and muscle recovery.

Designing an exercise routine for the 10-day transformation plays a significant role in maximizing the benefits of the program. By assessing your fitness level, setting clear goals, incorporating a variety of exercise modalities, considering time and intensity, prioritizing warm-up and cool-down, including strength training and core stability exercises, allowing for rest and recovery, and maintaining proper hydration and nutrition, you can create a well-rounded and effective exercise routine. Embrace the opportunity to empower your body and mind through regular physical activity, and let it complement the holistic transformation you are undergoing.

6.3 Incorporating movement into your daily life

In a sedentary world where technology often dominates our lives, it is crucial to prioritize movement and physical activity. Incorporating regular movement into our daily lives has numerous benefits for our physical, mental, and emotional well-being.

Regular movement is essential for maintaining physical health. It improves cardiovascular health, strengthens muscles and bones, and enhances flexibility and balance. Engaging in physical activity helps manage weight, reduces the risk of chronic diseases, and promotes overall vitality. By incorporating movement into our daily lives, we invest in our physical well-being and increase our longevity.

Movement has a profound impact on mental and emotional well-being. Engaging in physical activity releases endorphins, the "feel-good" hormones that elevate mood and reduce stress. Regular movement improves cognitive function, enhances focus and concentration, and boosts energy levels. It also promotes better sleep and helps alleviate symptoms of anxiety and depression. By incorporating movement, we enhance our mental and emotional well-being, fostering a positive outlook and improving overall quality of life.

Incorporating movement into our daily lives has a direct impact on our energy levels and productivity. Physical activity increases blood flow and oxygenation, improving brain function and mental clarity. It boosts energy levels, helping us feel more alert, focused, and motivated throughout the day. Regular movement also helps prevent fatigue and burnout, allowing us to be more productive and efficient in our daily tasks.

By incorporating movement into our daily lives, we create healthy habits that become a natural part of our routine. Consistency is key to reaping the benefits of physical activity. Making movement a regular practice helps establish a positive habit loop, where the desire to move becomes ingrained in our behavior. Over time, it becomes easier and more enjoyable to engage in regular physical activity.

Finding opportunities for movement is essential in our sedentary lifestyles. Incorporate physical activity into your daily routine by taking the stairs instead of the elevator, walking or biking to work, or engaging in active hobbies such as gardening, dancing, or sports. Incorporate short bursts of activity throughout the day, such as stretching breaks or brief walks during work breaks. Look for opportunities to move and make them a priority in your daily schedule.

Incorporating movement should be enjoyable and varied. Explore different forms of exercise and physical activities to find what suits your interests and preferences. Try activities such as yoga, dancing, swimming, hiking, or group fitness classes. Engage in activities that bring you joy and keep you motivated. Embracing variety and fun ensures that movement becomes a sustainable and enjoyable part of your daily life.

Set realistic goals and track your progress to stay motivated and accountable. Start with small, achievable goals and gradually increase intensity and duration as your fitness level improves. Use activity trackers or apps to monitor your daily steps, distance covered, or calories burned. Celebrate milestones and achievements to stay motivated and maintain a positive mindset.

Incorporating movement into our daily lives is essential for our overall well-being. By prioritizing physical activity, we enhance our physical health, boost mental and emotional well-being, increase energy levels, and create healthy habits. Finding opportunities for movement, embracing variety, and setting realistic goals ensure that physical activity becomes an enjoyable and sustainable part of our daily routines. Let us prioritize movement, embrace an active lifestyle, and reap the countless benefits it offers for our well-being and vitality.

CHAPTER SEVEN
Mindfulness and Stress Management

7.1 Understanding the impact of stress on health

In today's sedentary world, incorporating movement into your daily life is crucial for maintaining optimal health and well-being. Engaging in regular physical activity throughout the day goes beyond dedicated exercise sessions and encompasses the integration of movement into various aspects of your routine.

1. Break the Sedentary Cycle:

Sedentary behavior has become a prevalent issue in modern society, with many people spending prolonged periods sitting or engaging in activities that require minimal movement. Incorporating movement into your daily life helps break this sedentary cycle and counteracts the negative effects of prolonged sitting. Aim to reduce sedentary time by introducing frequent breaks and opportunities for movement throughout the day.

2. Embrace Active Transportation:

Opt for active transportation whenever possible. Choose walking or cycling instead of driving short distances. Use stairs instead of elevators or escalators. Incorporating active transportation not only increases your daily physical activity but also reduces carbon emissions and contributes to environmental sustainability.

3. Make Movement a Priority:

Prioritize movement by setting aside dedicated time for physical activity each day. Whether it's going for a brisk walk, practicing yoga, or engaging in a workout session, designate time to engage in structured exercise that aligns with your interests and goals. Making movement a priority ensures that it remains an integral part of your routine.

4. Integrate Movement into Daily Tasks:

Find opportunities to integrate movement into daily tasks and activities. For example, stand or pace while talking on the phone, do squats or lunges while brushing your teeth, or take short walking breaks during long periods of sitting. Look for creative ways to infuse movement into routine activities, making them more active and engaging.

5. Workstation Wellness:

If you have a sedentary job, prioritize workstation wellness. Incorporate ergonomic practices, such as using a standing desk, taking regular stretch breaks, and incorporating active movements like desk exercises or walking meetings. These strategies not only promote physical activity but also improve posture, reduce the risk of musculoskeletal issues, and enhance productivity.

6. Engage in Active Leisure:

Rather than spending leisure time in sedentary activities, choose active pursuits that bring you joy. Engage in hobbies like dancing, swimming, hiking, gardening, or playing a sport. Active leisure activities not only provide physical benefits but also contribute to mental and emotional well-being, offering an opportunity to unwind and enjoy life.

7. Set Activity Goals:

Set specific activity goals to ensure you are consistently incorporating movement into your daily life. Aim for a certain number of steps per day or set targets for active minutes. Use wearable fitness trackers or smartphone apps to monitor your progress and stay motivated. Gradually increase your goals over time to continue challenging yourself.

Benefits of Incorporating Movement

Incorporating movement into your daily life offers numerous benefits:

a. Improved Physical Fitness: Regular movement supports cardiovascular health, increases muscle strength and endurance, and enhances flexibility and mobility.

b. Weight Management: Incorporating movement helps maintain a healthy body weight by burning calories and promoting a balanced energy expenditure.

c. Enhanced Mental Well-being: Physical activity releases endorphins, reducing stress, anxiety, and symptoms of depression. It boosts mood, promotes relaxation, and improves overall mental well-being.

d. Increased Energy Levels: Engaging in regular movement increases energy levels, combats fatigue, and enhances productivity throughout the day.

e. Improved Cognitive Function: Physical activity stimulates brain function, enhances focus, memory, and cognitive abilities, and reduces the risk of age-related cognitive decline.

f. Long-Term Health Benefits: Regular movement reduces the risk of chronic diseases such as heart disease, type 2 diabetes, obesity, and certain types of cancer.

Incorporating movement into your daily life is essential for maintaining a healthy and active lifestyle. By breaking the sedentary cycle, embracing active transportation, prioritizing movement, integrating it into daily tasks, focusing on workstation wellness, engaging in active leisure, and setting activity goals, you can make movement a natural part of your routine. Embrace an active lifestyle, and reap the myriad benefits it offers for your physical, mental, and emotional well-being.

7.2 Practicing mindfulness and relaxation techniques

Stress has become a pervasive aspect of modern life, affecting individuals of all ages and backgrounds. While stress is a natural response to challenges, prolonged or chronic stress can have a detrimental impact on our overall health and well-being.

1. Physical Health Implications:

Stress has a significant impact on our physical health, manifesting in various ways:

a. Cardiovascular System: Chronic stress can lead to elevated blood pressure, increased heart rate, and the release of stress hormones, such as cortisol and adrenaline. Over time, this can contribute to the development of hypertension, heart disease, and an increased risk of stroke.

b. Immune System: Prolonged stress weakens the immune system, making individuals more susceptible to infections, illnesses, and autoimmune disorders. It can impair the body's ability to fight off pathogens and delay the healing process.

c. Digestive System: Stress can disrupt digestion, leading to gastrointestinal issues like stomach ulcers, acid reflux, irritable bowel syndrome (IBS), and appetite changes. Chronic stress can also contribute to unhealthy eating patterns, leading to weight gain or loss.

d. Sleep Disorders: Stress can interfere with sleep patterns, resulting in insomnia, difficulty falling asleep, or disrupted sleep. Inadequate sleep further compounds the effects of stress on overall health and well-being.

2. Mental and Emotional Well-being:

Stress profoundly affects mental and emotional well-being, influencing various aspects of our lives:

a. Anxiety and Depression: Chronic stress can contribute to the development or exacerbation of anxiety disorders and depression. Persistent feelings of worry, restlessness, irritability, and a lack of motivation are common symptoms.

b. Cognitive Function: Prolonged stress impairs cognitive function, including memory, concentration, and decision-making abilities. It can also lead to brain fog, difficulty focusing, and decreased productivity.

c. Mood and Emotional Stability: Stress can disrupt emotional stability, leading to mood swings, irritability, anger, and a decreased ability to cope with everyday challenges. It can also diminish overall life satisfaction and happiness.

d. Mental Disorders: Chronic stress is a risk factor for the development of mental disorders such as post-traumatic stress disorder (PTSD) and substance abuse disorders. It can exacerbate existing mental health conditions as well.

3. Behavioral and Lifestyle Factors:

Stress influences various behavioral and lifestyle factors, potentially leading to further health complications:

a. Unhealthy Coping Mechanisms: Individuals under stress may resort to unhealthy coping mechanisms such as overeating, substance abuse, smoking, or excessive alcohol consumption. These behaviors can have detrimental effects on physical and mental health.

b. Disrupted Sleep Patterns: Stress can disrupt sleep, leading to inadequate rest and an increased risk of sleep disorders. Sleep deprivation further exacerbates stress, creating a vicious cycle.

c. Reduced Physical Activity: Stress often leads to a decrease in physical activity, which negatively impacts overall fitness, cardiovascular health, and metabolism. This can contribute to weight gain, muscle loss, and decreased energy levels.

d. Social Withdrawal: Chronic stress can lead to social withdrawal, isolating individuals from social support networks. Lack of social connection can further contribute to feelings of loneliness, depression, and compromised mental well-being.

Understanding the profound impact of stress on health underscores the significance of managing and mitigating stress in our lives. By prioritizing stress management techniques, such as exercise, mindfulness, relaxation techniques, social support, and seeking professional help when needed, we can foster balance and well-being. Taking proactive steps to reduce stress not only improves our physical health but also promotes mental and emotional resilience, allowing us to lead healthier, more fulfilling lives.

7.3 Managing stress during the transformation process

Embarking on a transformation journey, whether it's for improving health, achieving personal goals, or pursuing a new lifestyle, can be both exciting and challenging. Stress often accompanies change, but it's essential to manage stress effectively to ensure a successful transformation.

Understanding the Impact of Stress:

Stress is a natural response to change, challenges, and demands. However, excessive and unmanaged stress can have detrimental effects on both physical and mental well-being. Chronic stress can lead to a weakened immune system, increased risk of chronic illnesses, impaired cognitive function, emotional instability, and decreased overall quality of life. Recognizing the impact of stress is the first step toward effectively managing it.

Self-Care and Stress Reduction Techniques:

Prioritizing self-care is crucial for managing stress during the transformation process. Engage in activities that promote relaxation, such as meditation, deep breathing exercises, yoga, or mindfulness practices. Incorporate regular physical activity into your routine, as exercise has been shown to reduce stress and boost mood. Take breaks and engage in hobbies or activities that bring you joy and provide a sense of calm.

Time Management and Prioritization:

Effective time management and prioritization are essential for reducing stress. Break down your transformation goals into smaller, manageable tasks. Create a schedule or to-do list that allows for balance and allocates time for self-care and relaxation. Avoid overloading your schedule and be realistic about what you can accomplish in a given timeframe. Delegate tasks when possible and learn to say no to additional commitments that may cause excessive stress.

Healthy Communication and Support Systems:

Effective communication and support systems play a significant role in managing stress. Share your transformation journey with trusted friends, family members, or support groups who can offer encouragement, understanding, and guidance. Seek support from professionals, such as therapists or coaches, who can provide valuable insights and strategies for managing stress and navigating challenges.

Mindfulness and Stress Reduction Practices:

Cultivating mindfulness and engaging in stress reduction practices can significantly reduce stress levels. Practice being present in the moment, focusing on the here and now rather than worrying about the future. Incorporate mindfulness techniques such as meditation, journaling, or gratitude exercises into your daily routine. These practices can help calm the mind, enhance self-awareness, and promote a sense of peace amidst the transformation process.

Healthy Coping Mechanisms:

Develop healthy coping mechanisms to manage stress effectively. Engage in activities that promote relaxation and provide a sense of comfort, such as reading, listening to music, engaging in creative outlets, or spending time in nature. Avoid unhealthy coping mechanisms like excessive alcohol or substance use, which can exacerbate stress and hinder the transformation process.

Flexibility and Adaptability:

Recognize that transformation journeys are not always linear, and setbacks or obstacles may arise. Embrace flexibility and adaptability as essential qualities for managing stress during the transformation process. Be open to adjusting your plans, seeking alternative solutions, and learning from setbacks. Embracing a growth mindset can help you navigate challenges with resilience and maintain a positive outlook.

Self-Reflection and Self-Compassion:

Engage in self-reflection to identify your stress triggers, patterns, and self-limiting beliefs. Practice self-compassion by treating yourself with kindness, understanding, and acceptance throughout the transformation process. Be patient with yourself and acknowledge that transformation takes time. Celebrate small victories and practice self-care regularly to nurture your well-being.

Managing stress during the transformation process is vital for ensuring a successful and sustainable journey. By understanding the impact of stress, practicing self-care, effective time management, fostering healthy communication, cultivating mindfulness, developing healthy coping mechanisms, embracing flexibility, and practicing self-compassion, you can navigate the transformation process with greater resilience, well-being, and a positive mindset. Remember, managing stress is not only crucial for the transformation itself but also for fostering a healthy and fulfilling life beyond it.

CHAPTER EIGHT
Quality Sleep for Vitality

8.1 The importance of sleep for overall well-being

Sleep is a fundamental aspect of human life, essential for maintaining overall well-being and functioning optimally. Despite its significance, sleep is often undervalued in today's fast-paced society.

1. Physical Restoration and Healing:

Sleep is a vital time for the body to restore and heal itself. During sleep, the body engages in essential processes such as tissue repair, muscle growth, and the release of hormones that regulate growth and repair. Sufficient sleep allows the body to recover from the day's activities, promoting physical health and resilience.

2. Cognitive Function and Mental Clarity

Sleep plays a crucial role in cognitive function and mental clarity. It enhances memory consolidation, learning, and problem-solving abilities. Adequate sleep supports attention, concentration, and decision-making skills, enabling individuals to perform at their best intellectually. On the other hand, sleep deprivation impairs cognitive function, leading to decreased productivity, poor focus, and difficulty in retaining information.

3. Emotional Well-being and Mood Regulation:

Sleep has a profound impact on emotional well-being and mood regulation. Sufficient sleep promotes emotional stability, resilience, and the ability to cope with stress. It helps regulate emotions, preventing mood swings, irritability, and heightened emotional reactivity. Conversely, sleep deprivation can contribute to mood disorders, increased anxiety, and a higher risk of developing mental health conditions.

4. Physical Health and Disease Prevention:

Quality sleep is closely linked to physical health and disease prevention. Chronic sleep deprivation has been associated with an increased risk of various health conditions, including obesity, diabetes, cardiovascular disease, and weakened immune function. Sleep plays a crucial role in maintaining a healthy weight, regulating blood sugar levels, and supporting the immune system's ability to fight off infections.

5. Hormonal Balance and Metabolic Health:

Sleep plays a vital role in hormonal balance and metabolic health. It helps regulate hormones involved in appetite control, such as leptin and ghrelin, thereby influencing hunger and satiety cues. Sufficient sleep supports a healthy metabolism and reduces the risk of weight gain and obesity. Inadequate sleep disrupts these hormonal pathways, increasing the likelihood of overeating and metabolic imbalances.

6. Enhancing Performance and Productivity:

Quality sleep directly impacts performance and productivity in various aspects of life. Whether it's academic, professional, or athletic pursuits, sleep plays a critical role in optimal functioning. Adequate sleep improves focus, attention, and problem-solving abilities. It enhances creativity and innovation, leading to higher levels of performance and productivity.

7. Immune System Function and Healing:

Sleep is essential for the proper functioning of the immune system. During sleep, the immune system releases cytokines, proteins that help combat inflammation, infection, and stress. Sufficient sleep strengthens the immune response, allowing the body to effectively fight off pathogens and recover from illnesses more rapidly.

8. Strategies for Prioritizing Sleep:

To prioritize sleep and reap its benefits, consider implementing the following strategies:

a. Establish a Consistent Sleep Schedule: Set a regular sleep routine, going to bed and waking up at the same time every day, even on weekends.

b. Create a Sleep-friendly Environment: Ensure your sleep environment is conducive to rest, with comfortable bedding, proper temperature, and minimal noise and light disturbances.

c. Practice Relaxation Techniques: Engage in relaxation activities before bed, such as reading, taking a warm bath, or practicing deep breathing exercises, to promote relaxation and prepare the mind and body for sleep.

d. Limit Stimulants and Electronic Devices: Avoid caffeine and stimulating substances close to bedtime. Minimize exposure to electronic devices that emit blue light, as it can interfere with the natural sleep-wake cycle.

e. Establish a Bedtime Routine: Develop a soothing routine before bed, such as listening to calming music, practicing meditation, or journaling, to signal to your body that it's time to wind down.

Sleep is a precious resource that should be prioritized for the sake of overall well-being and vitality. It plays a crucial role in physical health, cognitive function, emotional well-being, and productivity. By recognizing the importance of sleep, implementing strategies for quality sleep, and making it a priority in our daily lives, we can nurture our well-being and lead healthier, more fulfilling lives.

8.2 Establishing healthy sleep habits

Healthy sleep habits are essential for optimal well-being and overall health. However, in today's fast-paced world, many individuals struggle with sleep disturbances and irregular sleep patterns.

Understanding the Importance of Healthy Sleep Habits:

Healthy sleep habits are crucial for physical, mental, and emotional well-being. They contribute to better cognitive function, improved mood, enhanced immune function, and increased overall productivity. By prioritizing sleep and establishing healthy habits, individuals can experience a range of benefits that positively impact their daily lives.

Consistency is Key:

Consistency plays a pivotal role in establishing healthy sleep habits. The body's internal clock, known as the circadian rhythm, thrives on routine. Maintaining a consistent sleep schedule helps regulate the circadian rhythm, promoting better quality sleep and waking up feeling refreshed. Consistency also helps set the body's expectations for sleep, making it easier to fall asleep and wake up naturally.

Create a Sleep-friendly Environment:

Designing a sleep-friendly environment is essential for promoting restful nights. Keep the bedroom cool, dark, and quiet. Minimize noise distractions by using earplugs or white noise machines. Invest in a comfortable mattress, pillows, and bedding that support proper spinal alignment and help reduce discomfort during sleep.

Establish a Bedtime Routine:

Establishing a bedtime routine signals to the body that it's time to unwind and prepare for sleep. Engage in relaxing activities before bed, such as reading a book, taking a warm bath, or practicing gentle stretching or yoga. Avoid stimulating activities or electronic devices that emit blue light, as they can interfere with the natural sleep-wake cycle.

Limit Stimulants and Napping:

Avoid consuming stimulants close to bedtime, as they can disrupt sleep. Caffeine, nicotine, and alcohol can interfere with the quality and duration of sleep. Additionally, limit daytime napping to ensure you're sufficiently tired when it's time to sleep at night. If you do nap, keep it short (around 20-30 minutes) and avoid napping too close to your bedtime.

Create a Relaxing Bedtime Ritual:

Engaging in a relaxing bedtime ritual can help transition your mind and body into a state of relaxation. Consider incorporating activities such as journaling, practicing mindfulness or meditation, or listening to calming music or guided sleep meditation. These practices can help quiet the mind, reduce stress, and promote a sense of calm before sleep.

Regular Exercise and Exposure to Natural Light:

Regular exercise during the day promotes better sleep at night. Engage in moderate-intensity exercise, such as walking, jogging, or yoga, at least a few hours before bedtime. Exposure to natural light during the day is also beneficial for regulating the circadian rhythm and promoting a healthy sleep-wake cycle.

Monitor and Manage Stress:

Stress can significantly impact sleep quality and duration. Implement stress management techniques, such as deep breathing exercises, meditation, or engaging in relaxing hobbies, to help calm the mind and promote a peaceful state before sleep. Establishing a bedtime routine that includes stress reduction techniques can facilitate a smoother transition into sleep.

Establishing healthy sleep habits is crucial for maintaining overall well-being and vitality. By prioritizing consistency, creating a sleep-friendly environment, establishing a bedtime routine, limiting stimulants and napping, creating a relaxing bedtime ritual, incorporating regular exercise and exposure to natural light, and managing stress, individuals can cultivate restful and rejuvenating nights. Embrace the power of healthy sleep habits and experience the transformative effects they have on your daily life.

8.3 Optimizing your sleep environment

Creating an optimal sleep environment is crucial for achieving restful and rejuvenating nights of sleep. The sleep environment plays a significant role in promoting relaxation, minimizing disruptions, and ensuring a deep and uninterrupted sleep.

Darkness and Light Control:

Darkness is essential for promoting the production of melatonin, a hormone that regulates sleep-wake cycles. To optimize your sleep environment, invest in blackout curtains or blinds to block out external light sources such as streetlights or early morning sunlight. Consider using an eye mask if complete darkness is challenging to achieve. Additionally, minimize the use of electronic devices with bright screens before bed, as they emit blue light that can interfere with melatonin production.

Temperature and Air Quality:

Maintaining a comfortable temperature in your sleep environment is crucial for quality sleep. The ideal bedroom temperature typically falls between 60 to 67 degrees Fahrenheit (15 to 19 degrees Celsius). Experiment with different bedding materials and layers to find what keeps you comfortably cool or warm throughout the night. Good ventilation and fresh air circulation contribute to better air quality, so ensure proper ventilation in your bedroom. Consider using an air purifier if you live in an area with poor air quality.

Noise Reduction:

Excessive noise can disrupt sleep and prevent you from reaching deep, restorative sleep stages. Implement strategies to reduce noise disturbances in your sleep environment. Use earplugs or consider investing in white noise machines or fans that create a consistent and soothing background noise. Alternatively, use soft earphones and listen to calming sounds or music designed to promote sleep.

Comfortable Bedding and Mattress:

A comfortable and supportive mattress and bedding are crucial for optimizing your sleep environment. Invest in a high-quality mattress that aligns with your preferred sleep position and provides adequate support for your body. Experiment with different types of pillows to find the one that offers optimal neck and head support. Choose bedding materials that are soft, breathable, and appropriate for your climate to ensure comfort throughout the night.

Clutter-Free and Serene Atmosphere:

A clutter-free and serene atmosphere in your sleep environment promotes relaxation and calmness. Keep your bedroom clean and organized, as a cluttered space can contribute to a sense of unease and restlessness. Create a soothing ambiance by choosing calming colors for your bedroom decor, such as soft blues or earth tones. Consider incorporating elements of nature, such as plants or nature-inspired artwork, to enhance the tranquil atmosphere.

Technology-Free Zone:

To optimize your sleep environment, make your bedroom a technology-free zone. Remove or minimize the presence of electronic devices such as televisions, computers, or smartphones. These devices not only emit blue light that interferes with sleep but also can be a source of distractions and stimulate your mind. Instead, create a space that promotes relaxation, introspection, and rejuvenation.

Personalized Sleep Rituals:

Establishing personalized sleep rituals can enhance the sleep environment and signal your body that it's time to unwind and prepare for sleep. Engage in calming activities before bed, such as reading a book, practicing gentle stretching or yoga, taking a warm bath, or listening to soothing music. Establishing a consistent bedtime routine can help transition your mind and body into a state of relaxation and promote better sleep quality.

Optimizing your sleep environment is a key factor in ensuring restful and rejuvenating nights of sleep. By creating a dark, quiet, and comfortable sleep environment, controlling temperature and air quality, minimizing noise disruptions, maintaining a clutter-free and serene atmosphere, and establishing personalized sleep rituals, you can create the ideal haven for restful nights. Prioritize the optimization of your sleep environment, as it plays a vital role in supporting overall health, well-being, and a refreshed start to each day.

CHAPTER NINE
Building a Supportive Environment

9.1 Engaging family and friends in your health transformation

Embarking on a health transformation journey can be challenging, but having a strong support system can make all the difference. Family and friends play a vital role in our lives, and involving them in our health transformation can enhance motivation, accountability, and overall success.

Engaging family and friends in your health transformation journey can provide the motivation and encouragement needed to stay committed and focused. When loved ones understand your goals and aspirations, they can offer words of encouragement, celebrate your achievements, and provide the necessary push during challenging times. Their support can fuel your determination and reinforce your belief in your ability to succeed.

Involving family and friends in your health transformation journey creates a sense of accountability. Sharing your goals and progress with them adds a level of commitment to your efforts. Knowing that others are invested in your success can serve as a powerful motivator to stay on track. Regular check-ins, progress updates, and sharing milestones with loved ones can help hold you accountable and reinforce your dedication to your health goals.

Family and friends can provide crucial emotional support during your health transformation. They can empathize with your struggles, offer a listening ear, and provide a safe space for you to express your feelings. Having someone to share your triumphs, setbacks, and challenges with can alleviate stress, reduce feelings of isolation, and enhance overall well-being. Their understanding and empathy can help you navigate the ups and downs of your journey.

Engaging family and friends in your health transformation can lead to shared activities and the development of healthy habits together. Plan physical activities such as walks, hikes, or workout sessions that you can enjoy with your loved ones. Explore healthy recipes and cook meals together, fostering a supportive and nutritious eating environment. By involving your family and friends in these activities, you create a positive and health-focused social circle that reinforces your commitment to change.

Each person brings unique perspectives, experiences, and knowledge to the table. Engaging family and friends in your health transformation journey allows for knowledge exchange and learning opportunities. Share what you have learned about nutrition, exercise, or other aspects of your transformation process, and encourage your loved ones to do the same. This exchange of information can broaden everyone's understanding of health and wellness, creating a culture of continuous learning within your social circle.

Involving family and friends in your health transformation journey can have a ripple effect, inspiring them to prioritize their own well-being. By setting a positive example through your actions, commitment, and dedication to your health goals, you become a source of inspiration for others. Your transformation journey can encourage loved ones to embark on their own paths toward better health, creating a supportive and positive environment for everyone involved.

Effective communication is key to involving family and friends in your health transformation. Share your goals, progress, and challenges openly and honestly. Encourage your loved ones to express their thoughts, concerns, and ideas. Engage in open dialogue, listen actively, and be receptive to their input and suggestions. This collaboration fosters a sense of unity, strengthens relationships, and ensures that everyone feels valued and involved in the process.

Engaging family and friends in your health transformation journey can be a game-changer. Their support, motivation, and understanding can fuel your commitment, enhance accountability, and provide a solid foundation for success. By involving loved ones in your journey, you create a network of support, encouragement, and shared experiences. Embrace the power of connection, communicate openly, and foster a supportive environment that promotes health and well-being for all. Together, you can achieve your health goals and inspire positive change in each other's lives.

9.2 Overcoming challenges and barriers

Embarking on any transformative journey comes with its fair share of challenges and barriers. Whether it's improving one's health, pursuing personal goals, or making lifestyle changes, obstacles are inevitable. However, it is in overcoming these challenges that true growth and success are achieved.

The first step in overcoming challenges is recognizing their existence. Challenges can manifest in various forms, such as self-doubt, lack of motivation, time constraints, financial limitations, or external pressures. Identifying and acknowledging these obstacles allows us to develop strategies to address them effectively.

Cultivating a growth mindset is crucial when facing challenges and barriers. Embrace the belief that obstacles are opportunities for learning and growth rather than insurmountable roadblocks. Approach challenges with resilience, perseverance, and a willingness to adapt. View setbacks as temporary and focus on finding solutions and lessons that will propel you forward.

Clear goal setting and strategic planning are vital in overcoming challenges. Break down your larger goals into smaller, actionable steps that are more manageable and achievable. Develop a detailed plan that outlines the specific actions you need to take, along with timelines and milestones. This structured approach helps navigate challenges by providing a roadmap and ensuring progress is made, even in the face of obstacles.

It is essential to seek support from others when facing challenges and barriers. Surround yourself with individuals who believe in your goals and are willing to provide encouragement, guidance, and assistance when needed. Build a support network that includes friends, family, mentors, or like-minded individuals who can offer insights, share experiences, and provide motivation during challenging times.

Failure and setbacks are inevitable on any transformative journey. However, it is through these experiences that we learn, grow, and gain resilience. Embrace failure as a stepping stone to success rather than a definitive endpoint. Analyze setbacks objectively, identify lessons learned, and adjust your approach accordingly. Embracing a mindset of continuous improvement allows you to overcome barriers with newfound knowledge and determination.

Being flexible and adaptable is key to overcoming challenges and barriers. Recognize that the path to success is rarely linear and may require adjustments along the way. Stay open-minded and be willing to reassess and modify your strategies when faced with unexpected obstacles. Embrace change and view it as an opportunity for growth and new possibilities.

Prioritizing self-care and well-being is essential in navigating challenges. Take care of your physical, mental, and emotional health. Engage in activities that reduce stress, promote relaxation, and rejuvenate your energy. Nurture positive habits such as regular exercise, healthy eating, quality sleep, and self-reflection. Taking care of yourself equips you with the resilience and strength needed to overcome challenges effectively.

Celebrating small victories along the way is crucial in maintaining motivation and momentum. Recognize and acknowledge your progress, no matter how small. Each step forward, no matter how insignificant it may seem, is a testament to your resilience and determination. Celebrating these achievements boosts confidence, reinforces positive behaviors, and provides the motivation needed to overcome future challenges.

Overcoming challenges and barriers is an integral part of any transformative journey. By recognizing challenges, cultivating a growth mindset, setting clear goals, seeking support, embracing failure, staying flexible, prioritizing self-care, and celebrating victories, you can navigate obstacles with resilience and determination. Remember, it is in the face of challenges that true growth occurs, and success is realized. Embrace the journey, stay focused, and persevere, for it is through overcoming challenges that you will ultimately achieve your goals and aspirations.

9.3 Creating a sustainable healthy lifestyle beyond the 10-day program

Embarking on a 10-day program can jumpstart your journey towards a healthier lifestyle. However, the true measure of success lies in sustaining those positive changes beyond the program's duration. Creating a sustainable healthy lifestyle requires long-term commitment, mindful choices, and a shift in mindset.

Creating a sustainable healthy lifestyle requires a mindset shift from short-term fixes to long-term changes. Recognize that health is a lifelong journey and that consistency and dedication are key. Embrace the idea of making permanent lifestyle changes rather than temporary adjustments. This shift in mindset sets the foundation for sustainable habits that can be maintained over time.

Focus on establishing core habits that form the basis of your healthy lifestyle. Identify the key areas of your well-being, such as nutrition, exercise, sleep, stress management, and self-care. Develop sustainable habits within each of these areas that align with your values and preferences. For example, make whole foods and balanced meals a regular part of your diet, incorporate enjoyable physical activities into your routine, prioritize quality sleep, practice stress-reducing techniques, and engage in activities that promote self-care and relaxation.

Sustainable lifestyle changes are more likely to be successful when approached with gradual progression and small steps. Avoid overwhelming yourself with too many changes all at once. Instead, focus on making incremental improvements over time. Start with one or two specific habits and gradually incorporate additional changes as you become comfortable and confident. This approach allows for better adaptation and ensures that the changes become ingrained as lasting habits.

Surround yourself with a supportive environment that encourages and reinforces your healthy lifestyle choices. Seek the support of family, friends, or like-minded individuals who share similar goals. Engage in activities together, exchange ideas, and provide mutual encouragement. Consider joining fitness classes, support groups, or online communities that provide a sense of belonging and accountability.

Regularly evaluate your progress and make necessary adjustments to maintain sustainability. Reflect on what is working well and what areas may need improvement. Assess whether your current habits and routines are aligned with your long-term goals. Make adjustments to address any challenges or barriers that may arise along the way. Flexibility and adaptability are essential in ensuring the sustainability of your healthy lifestyle.

A sustainable healthy lifestyle involves continuous learning and exploration. Stay informed about current research, trends, and developments in the field of health and wellness. Explore new recipes, try different forms of exercise, and experiment with various stress management techniques. By embracing a mindset of continuous learning and exploration, you can discover what works best for you and adapt your lifestyle accordingly.

Be kind to yourself and practice self-compassion throughout your journey. Acknowledge that setbacks may happen, and it's okay to make mistakes along the way. Learn from them and use them as opportunities for growth. Be forgiving of yourself and avoid dwelling on past slip-ups. Remember that sustainable change is a lifelong process, and each day is an opportunity to make positive choices.

Creating a sustainable healthy lifestyle beyond the 10-day program requires a long-term commitment and a shift in mindset. By establishing core habits, taking gradual steps, building a supportive environment, regularly evaluating and adjusting, continuously learning, and practicing self-compassion, you can maintain your progress and enjoy lasting well-being. Embrace the journey as an ongoing process of growth and self-discovery, and let your commitment to a healthy lifestyle extend far beyond the initial program.

CHAPTER TEN
Celebrating Your Transformation

10.1 Recognizing achievements and milestones

In our pursuit of personal growth and success, it is crucial to acknowledge and celebrate our achievements and milestones along the way. Recognizing the progress we make on our journey not only boosts our self-confidence and motivation but also reinforces positive behaviors.

Recognizing achievements and milestones serves as a powerful source of motivation. Each milestone reached or goal accomplished validates our efforts and reinforces our belief in our abilities. Celebrating these accomplishments boosts self-confidence and encourages us to continue striving for further success. By acknowledging our achievements, we ignite the internal drive to push ourselves even further.

Recognizing achievements and milestones allows us to track our progress and reflect on our journey. It provides an opportunity to assess how far we have come and the challenges we have overcome. Reflecting on our achievements helps us gain a deeper understanding of our strengths, weaknesses, and areas for growth. It enables us to adjust our strategies and approach moving forward, based on the lessons learned from past successes.

Acknowledging achievements and milestones cultivates self-awareness and gratitude. It prompts us to be more mindful of our actions, decisions, and the impact they have on our lives. As we recognize our achievements, we develop a deeper appreciation for the effort, determination, and sacrifices we have made to reach our goals. Expressing gratitude for the opportunities, support, and resources that have contributed to our success further strengthens our sense of fulfillment and overall well-being.

Celebrating achievements and milestones reinforces positive behaviors and habits. When we recognize our progress, we reinforce the actions and decisions that led to that success. By acknowledging the positive impact of our efforts, we are more likely to continue practicing the behaviors that contributed to our achievements. This reinforcement builds positive habits and fosters a cycle of continuous growth and improvement.

Recognizing achievements and milestones strengthens our resilience and equips us to face future challenges. It serves as a reminder of our ability to overcome obstacles and persevere in the face of adversity. Celebrating our accomplishments during difficult times provides us with the motivation and inspiration needed to navigate challenges with confidence and determination. It reinforces our belief that we are capable of overcoming any obstacles that may come our way.

Recognizing achievements and milestones also allows us to share our success and inspire others. By celebrating our accomplishments, we create an opportunity to inspire and motivate those around us. Sharing our journey and the lessons we have learned along the way can encourage others to pursue their own goals and aspirations. Celebrating together builds a supportive community that uplifts and encourages personal growth in everyone involved.

There are various ways to recognize achievements and milestones. It can be as simple as acknowledging and praising oneself for a job well done. Additionally, sharing your success with trusted friends, family members, or mentors who have supported you throughout your journey can be empowering. Other ways to celebrate include setting aside dedicated time for self-reflection, treating yourself to a special reward or indulgence, or documenting your progress through journals or visual aids.

Recognizing achievements and milestones is an essential part of personal development and success. By acknowledging our progress, we cultivate motivation, enhance self-confidence, and reinforce positive behaviors. Celebrating our accomplishments allows us to reflect on our journey, express gratitude, and inspire others. Embrace the power of recognizing achievements and milestones on your path to growth, and let it fuel your continued pursuit of success and fulfillment.

10.2 Reflections on the 10-day journey

Embarking on a 10-day journey can be a transformative experience, offering an opportunity to make positive changes and create lasting habits. As the journey comes to an end, it is important to take the time to reflect on the lessons learned, the progress made, and the impact it has had on our lives.

The 10-day journey often brings about self-discovery and a heightened sense of self-awareness. Throughout the process, we become more attuned to our habits, emotions, and thought patterns. We gain insights into our strengths, weaknesses, and areas for growth. This increased self-awareness allows us to make more conscious choices and align our actions with our goals and values.

The 10-day journey provides an opportunity to challenge and transform our existing habits. By consciously implementing new practices and breaking free from old patterns, we create space for growth and change. Whether it is adopting healthier eating habits, incorporating regular exercise, practicing mindfulness, or managing stress more effectively, the journey encourages positive shifts that can extend beyond the initial program.

The journey often deepens our understanding of the mind-body connection. Through various practices such as mindful eating, exercise, and stress management techniques, we come to realize the profound impact our mental and emotional state has on our physical well-being. This awareness fosters a holistic approach to health and encourages us to prioritize self-care and balance in our daily lives.

The 10-day journey tests our resilience and strengthens our discipline. It requires commitment, consistency, and the willingness to overcome challenges and setbacks. As we navigate through the ups and downs, we develop a sense of resilience and determination. This newfound strength extends beyond the program, equipping us to face future obstacles with courage and perseverance.

The journey teaches us the value of celebrating small wins along the way. Each day presents an opportunity for progress, no matter how small. By acknowledging and appreciating these milestones, we cultivate a positive mindset and build momentum towards our goals. This practice of recognizing and celebrating small wins fosters a sense of accomplishment, boosting motivation and fueling further progress.

The 10-day journey serves as a catalyst for lifelong learning and growth. It opens the door to new knowledge, skills, and perspectives. As we delve into different aspects of health and well-being, we become curious and eager to expand our understanding. This thirst for knowledge propels us on a continuous journey of self-improvement and personal development beyond the initial program.

Reflection on the 10-day journey highlights the importance of integrating and sustaining the practices learned into our daily lives. As we evaluate the impact of the program, we identify which habits and practices resonate with us and align with our long-term goals. We prioritize incorporating these sustainable practices into our routines, ensuring that the positive changes made during the journey continue to shape our future.

Reflecting on the 10-day journey provides an opportunity to appreciate the transformation, growth, and valuable lessons gained along the way. It deepens our self-awareness, strengthens our discipline, and nurtures a holistic approach to well-being. By recognizing the impact of the journey and integrating sustainable practices, we set ourselves on a path of continued growth and a life filled with vitality, balance, and fulfillment.

10.3 Maintaining a vibrant and healthy life going forward

After experiencing a transformative journey towards a vibrant and healthy life, it is essential to maintain the progress and continue prioritizing well-being. Sustaining a vibrant and healthy life requires ongoing commitment, mindfulness, and a proactive approach to self-care.

Consistency is crucial in maintaining a vibrant and healthy life. Embrace the habits and practices that have contributed to your well-being during the journey. Make mindful choices in your daily life, focusing on nutrition, exercise, sleep, stress management, and self-care. Consistency creates a solid foundation for long-term success and ensures that your vibrant and healthy lifestyle becomes a sustainable reality.

Set realistic and achievable goals that align with your long-term vision of a vibrant and healthy life. These goals can include maintaining a specific weight, incorporating regular exercise, improving mental well-being, or pursuing new hobbies and interests. Personalize your goals based on your preferences, lifestyle, and values. By setting meaningful goals, you create a roadmap for sustained success and motivation.

Embrace a mindset of continuous learning and adaptation. Stay updated on the latest research, trends, and developments in health and wellness. Be open to exploring new approaches, refining your practices, and adjusting your routines based on new information or personal preferences.

Continually seek knowledge and be willing to adapt your habits to optimize your well-being.

Surround yourself with a supportive environment and build strong relationships that encourage your vibrant and healthy lifestyle. Seek the support of family, friends, or like-minded individuals who share similar goals. Engage in activities together, exchange ideas, and provide mutual encouragement. Create a network of support that fosters accountability, motivation, and a sense of belonging.

Prioritize self-care as an essential component of maintaining a vibrant and healthy life. Make time for activities that nourish your mind, body, and soul. Practice self-compassion, engage in hobbies you enjoy, and set boundaries to ensure a balanced lifestyle. Remember that self-care is not selfish; it is a necessary investment in your overall well-being.

Regularly evaluate your progress and reflect on your journey. Assess the effectiveness of your habits and routines. Identify areas where you can improve or adjust your approach. Celebrate your achievements and acknowledge any setbacks or challenges as opportunities for growth. Reflection allows you to fine-tune your strategies and reinforce the practices that contribute to your vibrant and healthy life.

Embrace a growth mindset that views challenges as opportunities for learning and improvement. Embrace failures and setbacks as valuable lessons rather than reasons to give up. Cultivate resilience, perseverance, and optimism in the face of obstacles. Adopting a growth mindset ensures that you continue to evolve and maintain a vibrant and healthy life, regardless of the challenges that come your way.

Maintaining a vibrant and healthy life beyond the transformative journey requires ongoing commitment and mindful choices. By prioritizing consistency, setting personalized goals, continuing to learn and adapt, cultivating a supportive environment, practicing self-care, engaging in regular evaluation and reflection, and embracing a growth mindset, you can sustain the positive changes and experience a life filled with vitality, balance, and well-being. Remember, the journey is ongoing, and your commitment to a vibrant and healthy life is a lifelong endeavor.

9 798396 056930